I0441116

Recipe:

Serving:

Prep Time:

Cook Time:

Temperature:

Ingredients:

Methods:

Wine Pairing:

From the Kitchen of:

Recipe: ______________________________

Serving: ____________ Prep Time: ____________

Cook Time: ____________ Temperature: ____________

Ingredients:

Methods:

Wine Pairing: ______________________________

From the Kitchen of: ______________________________

Recipe:

Serving:

Prep Time:

Cook Time:

Temperature:

Ingredients:

Methods:

Wine Pairing:

From the Kitchen of:

Recipe: ____________________

Serving: __________ Prep Time: __________

Cook Time: __________ Temperature: __________

Ingredients:

Methods:

Wine Pairing: ____________________

From the Kitchen of: ____________________

Recipe:

Serving:

Prep Time:

Cook Time:

Temperature:

Ingredients:

Methods:

Wine Pairing:

From the Kitchen of:

Recipe:

Serving:

Prep Time:

Cook Time:

Temperature:

Ingredients:

Methods:

Wine Pairing:

From the Kitchen of:

Recipe:

Serving:

Prep Time:

Cook Time:

Temperature:

Ingredients:

Methods:

Wine Pairing:

From the Kitchen of:

Recipe:

Serving:

Prep Time:

Cook Time:

Temperature:

Ingredients:

Methods:

Wine Pairing:

From the Kitchen of:

Recipe:

Serving:

Prep Time:

Cook Time:

Temperature:

Ingredients:

Methods:

Wine Pairing:

From the Kitchen of:

Recipe: ______________________

Serving: ____________ Prep Time: ____________

Cook Time: ____________ Temperature: ____________

Ingredients:

Methods:

Wine Pairing: ______________________

From the Kitchen of: ______________________

Recipe:

Serving:

Prep Time:

Cook Time:

Temperature:

Ingredients:

Methods:

Wine Pairing:

From the Kitchen of:

Recipe:

Serving:

Prep Time:

Cook Time:

Temperature:

Ingredients:

Methods:

Wine Pairing:

From the Kitchen of:

Recipe:

Serving:

Prep Time:

Cook Time:

Temperature:

Ingredients:

Methods:

Wine Pairing:

From the Kitchen of:

Recipe: ______________________

Serving: __________ Prep Time: __________

Cook Time: __________ Temperature: __________

Ingredients:

Methods:

Wine Pairing: ______________________

From the Kitchen of: ______________________

Recipe:

Serving:

Prep Time:

Cook Time:

Temperature:

Ingredients:

Methods:

Wine Pairing:

From the Kitchen of:

Recipe:

Serving:

Prep Time:

Cook Time:

Temperature:

Ingredients:

Methods:

Wine Pairing:

From the Kitchen of:

Recipe:

Serving:

Prep Time:

Cook Time:

Temperature:

Ingredients:

Methods:

Wine Pairing:

From the Kitchen of:

Recipe: ______________________________

Serving: ____________ Prep Time: ____________

Cook Time: ____________ Temperature: ____________

Ingredients:

Methods:

Wine Pairing: ______________________________

From the Kitchen of: ______________________________

Recipe:

Serving:

Prep Time:

Cook Time:

Temperature:

Ingredients:

Methods:

Wine Pairing:

From the Kitchen of:

Recipe:

Serving:

Prep Time:

Cook Time:

Temperature:

Ingredients:

Methods:

Wine Pairing:

From the Kitchen of:

Recipe:

Serving: Prep Time:

Cook Time: Temperature:

Ingredients:

Methods:

Wine Pairing:

From the Kitchen of:

Recipe:

Serving:

Prep Time:

Cook Time:

Temperature:

Ingredients:

Methods:

Wine Pairing:

From the Kitchen of:

Recipe:

Serving:

Prep Time:

Cook Time:

Temperature:

Ingredients:

Methods:

Wine Pairing:

From the Kitchen of:

Recipe:

Serving:

Prep Time:

Cook Time:

Temperature:

Ingredients:

Methods:

Wine Pairing:

From the Kitchen of:

Recipe:

Serving:

Prep Time:

Cook Time:

Temperature:

Ingredients:

Methods:

Wine Pairing:

From the Kitchen of:

Recipe:

Serving:

Prep Time:

Cook Time:

Temperature:

Ingredients:

Methods:

Wine Pairing:

From the Kitchen of:

Recipe:

Serving:

Prep Time:

Cook Time:

Temperature:

Ingredients:

Methods:

Wine Pairing:

From the Kitchen of:

Recipe:

Serving:

Prep Time:

Cook Time:

Temperature:

Ingredients:

Methods:

Wine Pairing:

From the Kitchen of:

Recipe:

Serving:

Prep Time:

Cook Time:

Temperature:

Ingredients:

Methods:

Wine Pairing:

From the Kitchen of:

Recipe:

Serving:

Prep Time:

Cook Time:

Temperature:

Ingredients:

Methods:

Wine Pairing:

From the Kitchen of:

Recipe:

Serving:

Prep Time:

Cook Time:

Temperature:

Ingredients:

Methods:

Wine Pairing:

From the Kitchen of:

Recipe:

Serving:

Prep Time:

Cook Time:

Temperature:

Ingredients:

Methods:

Wine Pairing:

From the Kitchen of:

Recipe:

Serving:

Prep Time:

Cook Time:

Temperature:

Ingredients:

Methods:

Wine Pairing:

From the Kitchen of:

Recipe:

Serving:

Prep Time:

Cook Time:

Temperature:

Ingredients:

Methods:

Wine Pairing:

From the Kitchen of:

Recipe:

Serving:

Prep Time:

Cook Time:

Temperature:

Ingredients:

Methods:

Wine Pairing:

From the Kitchen of:

Recipe:

Serving:

Prep Time:

Cook Time:

Temperature:

Ingredients:

Methods:

Wine Pairing:

From the Kitchen of:

Recipe:

Serving:

Prep Time:

Cook Time:

Temperature:

Ingredients:

Methods:

Wine Pairing:

From the Kitchen of:

Recipe:

Serving: | Prep Time:

Cook Time: | Temperature:

Ingredients: | Methods:

Wine Pairing:

From the Kitchen of:

Recipe:

Serving:

Prep Time:

Cook Time:

Temperature:

Ingredients:

Methods:

Wine Pairing:

From the Kitchen of:

Recipe:

Serving:

Prep Time:

Cook Time:

Temperature:

Ingredients:

Methods:

Wine Pairing:

From the Kitchen of:

Recipe:

Serving:

Prep Time:

Cook Time:

Temperature:

Ingredients:

Methods:

Wine Pairing:

From the Kitchen of:

Recipe:

Serving:

Prep Time:

Cook Time:

Temperature:

Ingredients:

Methods:

Wine Pairing:

From the Kitchen of:

Recipe:

Serving:

Prep Time:

Cook Time:

Temperature:

Ingredients:

Methods:

Wine Pairing:

From the Kitchen of:

Recipe:

Serving:

Prep Time:

Cook Time:

Temperature:

Ingredients:

Methods:

Wine Pairing:

From the Kitchen of:

Recipe:

Serving:

Prep Time:

Cook Time:

Temperature:

Ingredients:

Methods:

Wine Pairing:

From the Kitchen of:

Recipe:

Serving:

Prep Time:

Cook Time:

Temperature:

Ingredients:

Methods:

Wine Pairing:

From the Kitchen of:

Recipe:

Serving:

Prep Time:

Cook Time:

Temperature:

Ingredients:

Methods:

Wine Pairing:

From the Kitchen of:

Recipe:

Serving:

Prep Time:

Cook Time:

Temperature:

Ingredients:

Methods:

Wine Pairing:

From the Kitchen of:

Recipe:

Serving:

Prep Time:

Cook Time:

Temperature:

Ingredients:

Methods:

Wine Pairing:

From the Kitchen of:

Recipe:

Serving:

Prep Time:

Cook Time:

Temperature:

Ingredients:

Methods:

Wine Pairing:

From the Kitchen of:

Recipe:

Serving:

Prep Time:

Cook Time:

Temperature:

Ingredients:

Methods:

Wine Pairing:

From the Kitchen of:

Recipe:

Serving:

Prep Time:

Cook Time:

Temperature:

Ingredients:

Methods:

Wine Pairing:

From the Kitchen of:

Recipe:

Serving:

Prep Time:

Cook Time:

Temperature:

Ingredients:

Methods:

Wine Pairing:

From the Kitchen of:

Recipe:

Serving:

Prep Time:

Cook Time:

Temperature:

Ingredients:

Methods:

Wine Pairing:

From the Kitchen of:

Recipe:

Serving:

Prep Time:

Cook Time:

Temperature:

Ingredients:

Methods:

Wine Pairing:

From the Kitchen of:

Recipe:

Serving: Prep Time:

Cook Time: Temperature:

Ingredients:

Methods:

Wine Pairing:

From the Kitchen of:

Recipe:

Serving:

Prep Time:

Cook Time:

Temperature:

Ingredients:

Methods:

Wine Pairing:

From the Kitchen of:

Recipe:

Serving:

Prep Time:

Cook Time:

Temperature:

Ingredients:

Methods:

Wine Pairing:

From the Kitchen of:

www.ingramcontent.com/pod-product-compliance
Lightning Source LLC
Chambersburg PA
CBHW071247280526
45788CB00004B/1622
* 9 7 8 1 0 9 8 8 2 0 1 7 6 *